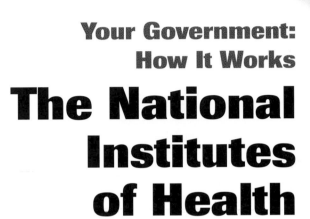

Your Government:
How It Works

The National Institutes of Health

Rich Mintzer

Chelsea House Publishers
Philadelphia

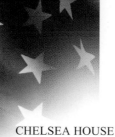

CHELSEA HOUSE PUBLISHERS
Editor in Chief Sally Cheney
Director of Production Kim Shinners
Creative Manager Takeshi Takahashi
Manufacturing Manager Diann Grasse

Staff for THE NATIONAL INSTITUTES OF HEALTH
Editor Colleen Sexton
Production Assistant Jaimie Winkler
Picture Researcher Jaimie Winkler
Series Designers Keith Trego, Takeshi Takahashi
Cover Designer Takeshi Takahashi
Layout 21st Century Publishing and Communications, Inc.

The Chelsea House World Wide Web address is
http://www.chelseahouse.com

First Printing
1 3 5 7 9 8 6 4 2

Library of Congress Cataloging-in-Publication Data

Mintzer, Rich.
    National Institutes of Health / by Rich Mintzer.
      p. cm.—(Your Government: How It Works)
Summary: Presents an overview of the history of infectious disease
epidemics in the United States, as well as the history of the National
Institutes of Health, the structure and role of that institution, and
current major health concerns that are its focus.
Includes bibliographical references and index.
    ISBN 0-7910-6793-9
    1. National Institutes of Health (U.S.)—Juvenile literature.
[1.National Institutes of Health (U.S.)] I. Title. II. Series.
RA11.D6 M55 2002
362.1'0973—dc21
                                                        2002000043

Dedication: Thank you to Victoria A. Harden, Ph.D., NIH Historian
and Director of the Dewitt Stetten, Jr. Museum of Medical
Research, for her assistance in preparing this book.

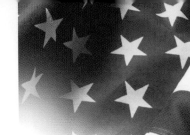

Contents

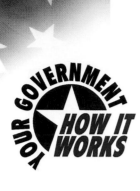

YOUR GOVERNMENT
HOW IT WORKS

Introduction

Government: Crises of Confidence

Arthur M. Schlesinger, jr.

FROM THE START, Americans have regarded their government with a mixture of reliance and mistrust. The men who founded the republic understood the importance of government. "If men were angels," observed the 51st Federalist Paper, "no government would be necessary." But men are not angels. Because human beings are subject to wicked as well as to noble impulses, government was deemed essential to assure freedom and order.

The American revolutionaries, however, also knew that government could become a source of injury and oppression. The men who gathered in Philadelphia in 1787 to write the Constitution therefore had two purposes in mind: They wanted to establish a strong central authority and to limit that central authority's capacity to abuse its power.

To prevent the abuse of power, the Founding Fathers wrote two basic principles into the Constitution. The principle of federalism divided power between the state governments and the central authority. The principle of the separation of powers subdivided the central authority itself into three branches—the executive, the legislative, and the judiciary—so that "each may be a check on the other."

YOUR GOVERNMENT: HOW IT WORKS examines some of the major parts of that central authority, the federal government. It explains how various officials, agencies, and departments operate and explores the political organizations that have grown up to serve the needs of government.

The federal government as presented in the Constitution was more an idealistic construct than a practical administrative structure. It was barely functional when it came into being.

This was especially true of the executive branch. The Constitution did not describe the executive branch in any detail. After vesting executive power in the president, it assumed the existence of "executive departments" without specifying what these departments should be. Congress began defining their functions in 1789 by creating the Departments of State, Treasury, and War.

President Washington, assisted by Secretary of the Treasury Alexander Hamilton, equipped the infant republic with a working administrative structure. Congress also continued that process by creating more executive departments as they were needed.

Throughout the 19th century, the number of federal government workers increased at a consistently faster rate than did the population. Increasing concerns about the politicization of public service led to efforts—bitterly opposed by politicians—to reform it in the latter part of the century.

The 20th century saw considerable expansion of the federal establishment. More importantly, it saw growing impatience with bureaucracy in society as a whole.

The Great Depression during the 1930s confronted the nation with its greatest crisis since the Civil War. Under Franklin Roosevelt, the New Deal reshaped the federal government, assigning it a variety of new responsibilities and greatly expanding its regulatory functions. By 1940, the number of federal workers passed the 1 million mark.

Critics complained of big government and bureaucracy. Business owners resented federal regulation. Conservatives worried about the impact of paternalistic government on self-reliance, on community responsibility, and on economic and personal freedom.

When the United States entered World War II in 1941, government agencies focused their energies on supporting the war effort. By the end of World War II, federal civilian employment had risen to 3.8 million. With peace, the federal establishment declined to around 2 million in 1950. Then growth resumed, reaching 2.8 million by the 1980s.

A large part of this growth was the result of the national government assuming new functions such as: affirmative action in civil rights, environmental protection, and safety and health in the workplace.

Some critics became convinced that the national government was a steadily growing behemoth swallowing up the liberties of the people. The 1980s brought new intensity to the debate about government growth. Foes of Washington bureaucrats preferred local government, feeling it more responsive to popular needs.

But local government is characteristically the government of the locally powerful. Historically, the locally powerless have often won their human and constitutional rights by appealing to the national government. The national government has defended racial justice against local bigotry, upheld the Bill of Rights against local vigilantism, and protected natural resources from local greed. It has civilized industry and secured the rights of labor organizations. Had the states' rights creed prevailed, perhaps slavery would still exist in the United States.

Americans are still of two minds. When pollsters ask large, spacious questions—Do you think government has become too involved in your lives? Do you think government should stop regulating business?—a sizable majority opposes big government. But when asked specific questions about the practical work of government—Do you favor Social Security? Unemployment compensation? Medicare? Health and safety standards in factories? Environmental protection?—a sizable majority approves of intervention.

We do not like bureaucracy, but we cannot live without it. We need its genius for organizing the intricate details of our daily lives. Without bureaucracy, modern society would collapse. It would be impossible to run any of the large public and private organizations we depend on without bureaucracy's division of labor and hierarchy of authority. The challenge is to keep these necessary structures of our civilization flexible, efficient, and capable of innovation.

More than 200 years after the drafting of the Constitution, Americans still rely on government but also mistrust it. These attitudes continue to serve us well. What we mistrust, we are more likely to monitor. And government needs our constant attention if it is to avoid inefficiency, incompetence, and arbitrariness. Without our informed participation, it cannot serve us individually or help us as a people to attain the lofty goals of the Founding Fathers.

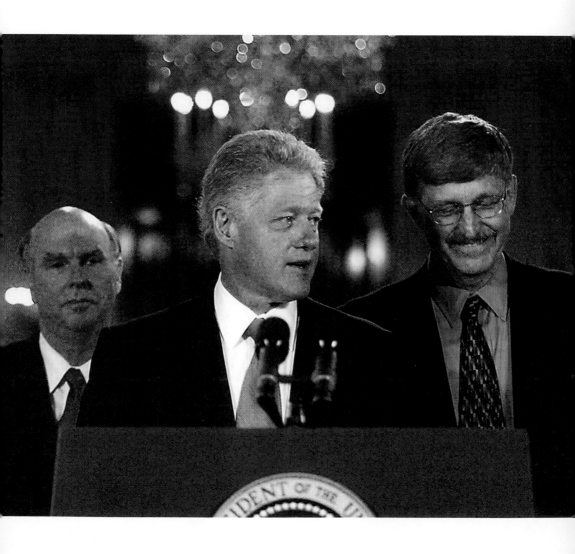

CHAPTER 1

Better Health for Everyone

ON THE MORNING of June 26, 2000, a crowd of U.S. government officials, foreign ambassadors, scientists, and journalists gathered in the East Room of the White House in Washington, D.C. They were there to mark a historic event. President Bill Clinton stepped to a podium and announced that an international team of scientists had completed the first survey of the entire human **genome,** the genetic blueprint for a human being. Calling it "the most important, most wondrous map ever produced by humankind," President Clinton congratulated those who had broken the genetic code.

This landmark achievement had its beginnings in 1944, when scientists Oswald Avery, Maclyn McCarty, and Colin McLeod determined that DNA is hereditary material. DNA, which stands for deoxyribonucleic acid, is a **molecule** found in every living **cell.** It is the substance that makes up genes, which determine an organism's characteristics. An organism's complete set of DNA is a genome.

In 1953, young scientists James Watson and Francis Crick discovered the double helix structure of DNA, a breakthrough that led to increased genetic research during the 20th century. In 1961, Marshall Nirenberg, the first government scientist to win a Nobel Prize, deciphered the code in DNA's double helix and showed how the code directed the construction of proteins in each cell. By the 1970s, scientists were talking about the possibility of decoding the entire human genome. In 1989, under Watson's leadership, the National Center for Human Genome Research (later renamed the National Human Genome Research Institute) was established as part of the National Institutes of Health. And in 1990, the organization helped launch the Human Genome Project, an international effort to discover the thousands of human genes and make them available for further biological study. They would also work to determine the DNA **sequences** of these genes.

More than 1,000 researchers from six nations were dedicated to the project. Dr. Francis Collins led the effort, which soon was accompanied by the work of scientists at Celera Genomics, a private-sector business headed by Dr. Craig Venter. Their efforts, along with the development of new technologies, enabled the Human Genome Project to move forward rapidly. The completion of the first "rough draft" of the human genome in 2001 was a year ahead of schedule. The project's leaders predict that a high-quality DNA reference sequence—the final goal of the project—will be available in 2003, two years earlier than originally planned.

Scientists, businesses, and government leaders around the world have envisioned the staggering number of benefits that the completion of this project will bring to humankind. Scientists will be able to more easily diagnose genetic diseases, including Alzheimer's disease and some

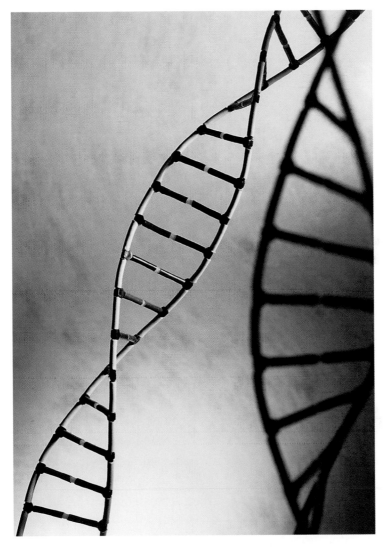

This model shows the double helix structure of DNA, a molecule found in every living cell. DNA directs the way that cells and organisms grow and reproduce.

cancers. They will be able to create more effective drugs. They will possibly even be able to find methods to prevent people from developing genetic diseases in the first place. And on a broader scale, they may gain a new understanding of human evolution. As President Clinton noted on that historic June day in 2001, the efforts of the scientists who worked on the Human Genome Project will "lead to a new era of molecular medicine, an era that will bring new ways to prevent, diagnose, treat, and cure disease."

The Human Genome Project is just one of many undertakings that fulfill the mission of the government-funded National Institutes of Health (NIH): to uncover new knowledge that will lead to better health for everyone. This mission is rooted in the U.S. Constitution, which states that one of the government's roles is to promote the general welfare of the people. Americans look to their government for health research, vital statistics on health, and control of contagious diseases. The NIH is one of eight health agencies of the Public Health Service, a part of the U.S. Department of Health and Human Services.

Disease in America

Diseases and the search for their prevention, treatments, and cures, have long been part of America's history. As far back as the early 1600s, there were outbreaks of **contagious** diseases on American soil. Even the original 105 settlers who made their home in Jamestown, Virginia, in 1607 were reduced to just 32 people in less than a year because of the spread of disease. Contact with animals, unclean drinking water, and exposure to unknown types of plants all caused the spread of illness among the early European settlers. And these diseases often spread to the American Indian population.

After one person contracted a disease, it spread from person to person very quickly. In a matter of a few weeks, an entire town could become sick, and there were not enough doctors, blankets, or supplies to help care for the ill. To make matters worse, much of America's population in the 1600s was in the northeastern part of the country, where cold, harsh winters made it especially difficult to keep patients healthy.

The rapid spread of a serious illness is called an epidemic. The history of American health is, unfortunately, filled with epidemics. Because an epidemic spreads quickly and the research for treatment or prevention takes time, it is very difficult to stop. Sometimes it takes years to find

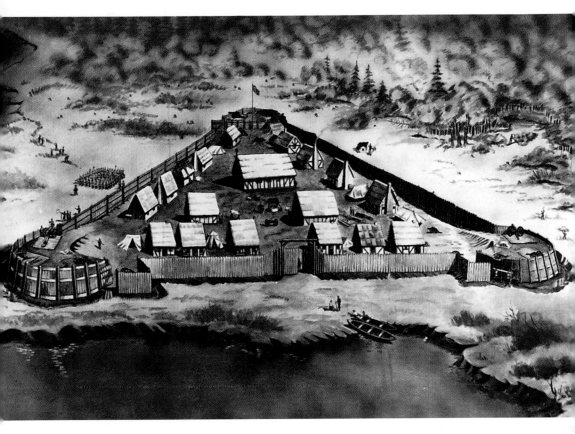

a **vaccine,** a treatment, or a cure for the disease causing the epidemic.

U.S. Epidemics

One of the earliest and most deadly epidemics to infect America was a tropical disease called yellow fever, which was brought to this country by settlers from South America. The disease, which is carried by mosquitoes, appeared as early as 1690. Symptoms include a high fever, chills, vomiting, and muscle aches. The disease affects the liver and other internal organs. An infected person's skin often turns yellow, a characteristic that gave the disease its name. Yellow fever spread through Philadelphia, Pennsylvania, in 1793, killing one of every ten people. Another yellow fever epidemic in the 1850s

In less than one year, diseases killed nearly two-thirds of the colonists at Jamestown, Virginia, which was established as America's first permanent settlement in 1607.

Certain mosquitoes can carry the yellow fever virus. When the mosquito bites a person who has yellow fever, the virus enters the insect's body. The mosquito's bite can then infect other people.

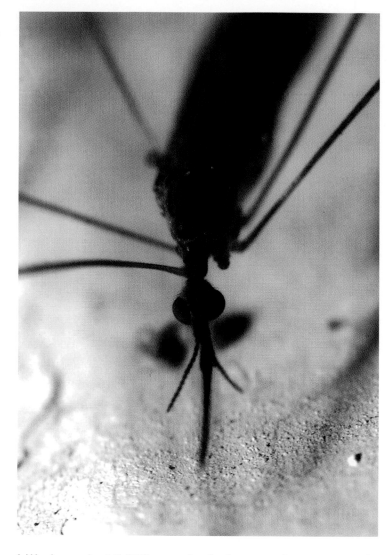

killed nearly 10,000 people during one hot summer in New Orleans, Louisiana, alone. It wasn't until 1937 that a South African scientist named Max Theiler invented a vaccine that helped eliminate the disease in most areas of the world.

Smallpox is one of the most dangerous diseases in history. This deadly disease, which is caused by a **virus** called variola, existed for thousands of years and killed millions of people. A high fever and a rash characterize

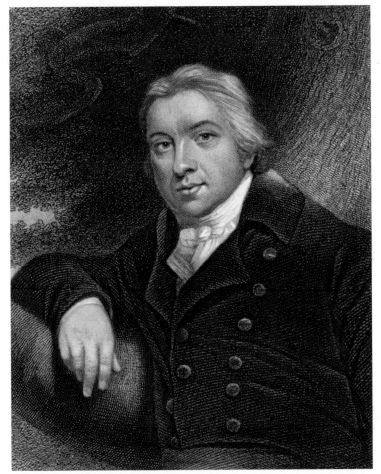

In 1796, British physician Edward Jenner developed the first vaccine, a means of preventing the contagious and deadly disease smallpox.

smallpox, which is highly contagious. In the United States, smallpox epidemics broke out sporadically from the 1600s through the early 1900s.

In 1796, British scientist Dr. Edward Jenner developed the first vaccine from cowpox, a mild skin disease that primarily affects cows. For many years, American scientists spent time researching ways to improve the vaccine. Years later, one of the jobs given to the NIH was to make sure the vaccines being produced from these animals were safe for humans. NIH scientists did research to test how well the vaccines worked and looked for any **side effects**.

It took more than 100 years for scientists to develop a vaccine that could be used worldwide. The World Health Organization announced in 1980 that smallpox had been eradicated. It became the first and only disease that humans eliminated from nature. Two known samples of the smallpox virus are kept in laboratories in Russia and the United States. Because experts believe it is possible that smallpox could be used deliberately as a biological weapon, the United States began to develop and store the vaccine in 2000.

Another epidemic that swept across America was influenza, commonly referred to as "the flu." Today, we treat the flu by resting, drinking liquids, and perhaps taking medications. But when the virus appeared in Virginia in 1793, the disease spread quickly, killing 500 people in less than a month. Influenza epidemics returned several times throughout the 1800s, but hit America hardest in 1918 during World War I (1914–1918). In fact, more people were hospitalized with influenza that year than were injured in the war.

The Public Health Service, which oversaw the laboratory that later became the NIH, worked hard to stop influenza from spreading. Doctors encouraged the army to keep the many infected soldiers away from civilians. They also tried to warn people about the early signs of influenza, which include a high fever, a sore throat, sweating, a headache, and an overall feeling of weakness. But their warnings could not stop the spread of the disease, and people in many cities fell ill with influenza.

The government provided the Public Health Service with money to hire more than 1,000 doctors and 700 nurses to help treat the growing number of patients. There were already many doctors and nurses treating soldiers and some had become ill themselves. Many of the research doctors who were working for the Public Health Service trying to find a cure had to leave their laboratories to care for sick patients. By the time the epidemic had finally disappeared in 1919, more than 500,000 people across the country, from New York City to San Francisco, had died from influenza.

A devastating epidemic of poliomyelitis, or polio, struck the New York area in 1916, and the illness flared up often throughout the country during the next 40 years. In serious cases, the polio virus may attack the nerve cells in the brain and spinal cord, leaving victims—often young children—paralyzed or disabled. Polio epidemics crippled or killed thousands of people in the United States. In 1952 alone, nearly 58,000 people became ill with the dreaded disease.

Researchers worked long and hard to develop a vaccine that would protect people from the polio virus. In 1952, American scientist Dr. Jonas Salk announced that he had created a vaccine that prevented polio. Trials of the vaccine showed that it did indeed work, and children worldwide began to be vaccinated. Shortly after it was first used, 200 people who had taken the vaccine became ill with polio, and the public thought that the vaccine was not working. Officials found, however, that a drug company had made a bad batch of the vaccine. This incident forced the NIH and other organizations to tighten up their rules about the safe production of vaccines by drug companies. Later, NIH scientists selected an oral polio vaccine created by Dr. Albert Sabin that was considered a better version of the original. Dr. Ruth Kirschstein, one of the scientists who had recommended the Sabin vaccine, then developed safety standards for its use.

From the 1950s, when the polio epidemic ended, until the early 1980s, the United States was free of the most deadly types of epidemics. Then the first signs of HIV, the virus that causes acquired immunodeficiency syndrome (AIDS), appeared. HIV, which stands for human immunodeficiency virus, can severely damage the

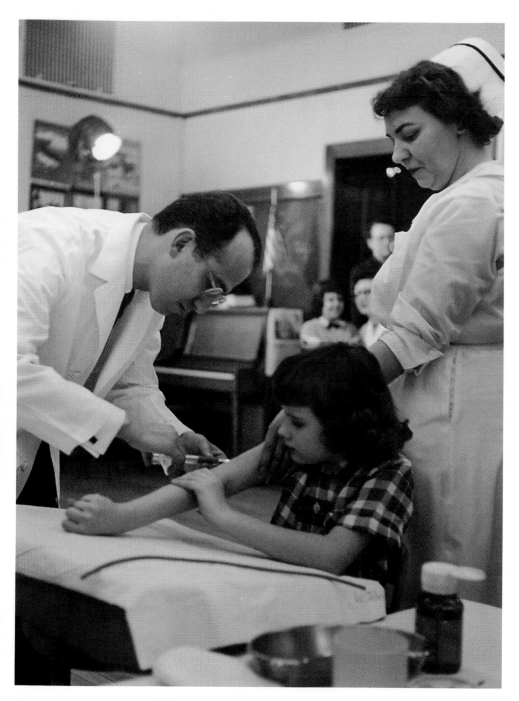

American scientist Jonas Salk vaccinates a girl against polio, a disease that can attack the brain and spinal cord. Salk developed the vaccine in 1952.

immune system, the body's main defense against disease. AIDS, the life-threatening stage of infection for people with HIV, has killed millions of people worldwide. HIV is transmitted through sexual intercourse or through direct contact with infected blood. It can also be passed from a mother to her unborn child. Scientists have developed treatments for HIV, but no cure has yet been found. The NIH created the Office of AIDS Research to coordinate planning and budgeting, as well as set priorities, for AIDS research at the various institutes that make up the NIH.

These epidemics—as well as cancer, heart disease, and other health conditions—have led many American scientists to dedicate their time to conducting experiments in laboratories. They have often found success. Many serious illnesses are now easy to treat. Other illnesses still have researchers working hard to find treatments and cures. Fueled by their mission of better health for everyone, the NIH is playing an important role in this research and in the health of people across the nation and worldwide.

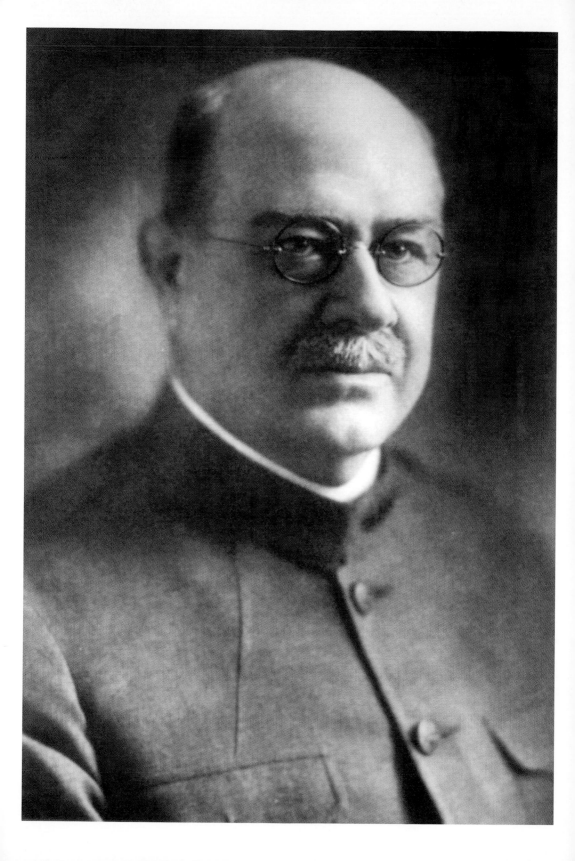

CHAPTER 2

The History of the NIH

TODAY, THE NIH is involved in thousands of research projects. Scientists use the latest microscopes and computers to help make amazing new discoveries. They research hundreds of illnesses and test many new medications and treatments every year. The influence of the NIH is especially astounding when you consider that it was just over 100 years ago that a young scientist in a one-room laboratory started this expansive organization.

Small Beginnings

As far back as the 1870s, scientists in Europe were studying **microscopic organisms** to find the causes of **infectious** diseases. Microscopes had been around for nearly 200 years, but scientists did not have the means to test the idea that tiny organisms too small to see with the naked eye could carry disease from one person to another.

Doctors and scientists in the United States were keeping a close eye on the research going on in Europe.

In 1887, officials at the Marine Hospital Service in New York City, which provided medical care to merchant seamen, decided it was time to open a research laboratory to study these microscopic organisms. They gave a young physician named Joseph Kinyoun this responsibility. Kinyoun had earned his medical degree at New York University in 1882. At the young age of 27, Kinyoun became the founder and director of this new laboratory, which he called a "laboratory of **hygiene**" to indicate that its purpose was to focus on public health. Shortly after starting the laboratory, he studied in Europe under the famous German bacteriologist Robert Koch.

It was in his new laboratory that Kinyoun identified the **bacteria** that caused cholera, a disease that people contracted by drinking water that wasn't clean or by eating fish from rivers that were polluted. He worked with doctors in the hospital who believed that their patients had cholera. Kinyoun's research proved that the doctors were correct. He was able to match the organism that he saw under his microscope to samples taken from the patient. His discovery showed that studying microscopic organisms could help doctors be certain which illness a patient had. But the microscopes of the time limited the diseases that could be tested. Although Kinyoun worked on many experiments related to yellow fever, the virus that caused the disease was too small to be seen through his light microscope. It wasn't until 1930, with the development of the electron microscope, that scientists were able to identify very small bacteria and viruses.

A Government Research Center

Kinyoun's laboratory became known as the Hygienic Laboratory, and in 1891 it was moved to Washington, D.C.

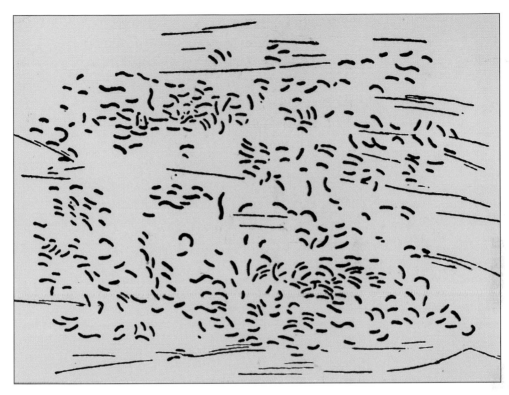

During the next 10 years, Kinyoun continued to operate the lab alone. Then in 1901, Congress designated $35,000 for construction of a new building for the laboratory. There, they said, scientists would study "infectious and contagious diseases and matters pertaining to the public health." This declaration was the first time Congress mentioned the laboratory in a law.

This drawing from the late 1800s shows how the cholera bacteria looked to early scientists under a microscope.

In 1902, two years before the Hygienic Laboratory moved into its new building, Congress passed two acts that helped launch the facility as a government research center. First they changed the name of the Marine Hospital Service to the Public Health and Marine Hospital Service and also added special divisions of chemistry, pharmacology, and zoology. The second piece of legislation was the Biologics Control Act. It gave the laboratory responsibility for supervising the production of vaccines and other medicines to make sure they were safe for public use. By 1907, scientists had established production standards and had started issuing licenses to companies that made the drugs.

Another name change came in 1912, when the organization became known as the Public Health Service (PHS). At this time, Congress authorized the laboratory to begin doing research on non-contagious diseases. Scientists still kept watch over the production of medicines and vaccines to make sure they were safe. They also conducted research on the possible positive effects of vitamins on people and even studied the negative effects of pollution in rivers and streams. If something affected the health of the American people, the PHS studied it.

The Ransdell Act

The PHS grew throughout the 1920s. But adding more researchers and buying better equipment meant spending more money. By the end of the 1920s, the United States had entered into the Great Depression. Many people had lost money in the stock market, and others were losing their jobs. The government was focused on recovering from this economic disaster, and there was not much money available for the PHS. At the same time, health concerns were growing because living conditions were increasingly poor and people were not eating well.

Meanwhile, a group of scientists who had worked for the government during World War I wanted to conduct research that would apply knowledge in chemistry to medicine. They had been working without much luck to obtain funding from wealthy individuals to open a private-sector institute. The scientists contacted Senator Joseph Ransdell of Louisiana in search of federal funding. Ransdell proposed legislation that would join this group of scientists with the PHS. The PHS would receive money and would grant funding for the scientists' research. In 1930, Congress passed the Ransdell Act, which changed the laboratory's name to the National Institute of Health.

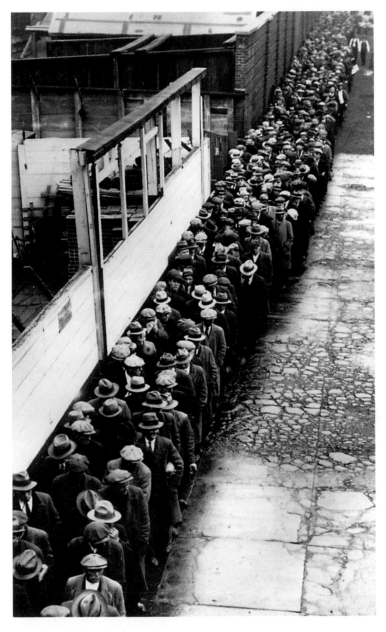

During the Great Depression of the 1930s, many people were homeless and jobless. Public health was a great concern at this time, but there was little money to support it.

By 1937, federal funding had also established the National Cancer Institute to conduct research on cancer, a growing health concern in the United States. The National Cancer Institute officially became part of the NIH in 1944.

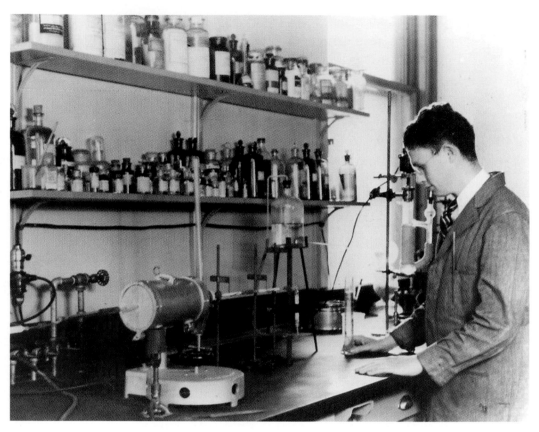

A lab technician works in an NIH facility in 1937.

War and Growth

During World War II (1939–1945), NIH scientists focused their attention on war-related problems. For example, there were many factories making weapons for the war. The NIH worked to make sure factory workers were protected so that their health and safety were not in danger. Factory workers began wearing protective suits to prevent injuries when they were working with dangerous weapons or chemicals. The work of the NIH during the war helped to improve working conditions for more than 300,000 workers in these weapons factories.

During these years, the NIH also worked to create vaccines to fight diseases that U.S. soldiers were contracting while fighting overseas. Wars were often the cause for spreading diseases, as soldiers had to survive in damp, cold, and dirty conditions. They often brought the diseases back home and spread them to civilians. The NIH helped prepare vaccines to prevent soldiers from getting yellow fever and other diseases.

As the war ended, the NIH began a period of growth. In 1948, the organization's name became plural, changing to the National Institutes of Health. By this time, the NIH's annual budget had expanded to more than $24 million, and the organization included six institutes. After World War II, Congress gave the NIH authority to award grants to aid research at universities. Congress also gave the NIH another mission: to conduct **clinical research.** At Warren Grant Magnuson Clinical Center, a hospital that opened in 1953, researchers and doctors began working together closely to develop medical treatments. Patients in the hospital were there to take part in research experiments. Government officials watched over the research to make sure that patients were not harmed.

The NIH experienced tremendous growth in the 1950s and 1960s, a period considered the golden years of the agency. By 1968, the NIH's annual budget had risen to more than $1 billion. The scope of the NIH's influence grew as more institutes were established. By 1970, the NIH included 15 institutes and centers. During these two decades, the NIH became a true leader in scientific research, spurred on by the development of new technologies.

The Modern NIH

By the end of the 1960s, **inflation** and new health programs such as Medicare and Medicaid began to eat into the funding available to the NIH. Scientists debated over which studies should receive more research money. Some scientists felt it was more important to study the human body in general, hoping to find ways to prevent many illnesses. Other scientists thought it was more important

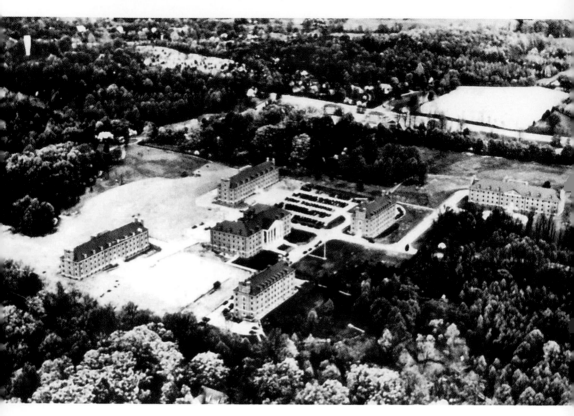

This aerial photograph shows the NIH campus in Bethesda, Maryland, in the 1940s, a time of great growth for the organization.

to study a specific disease and seek out a cure. In response to the latter idea, Congress focused on funding for two deadly diseases—cancer and heart disease—in the early 1970s. On the other hand, when HIV and AIDS reached crisis levels beginning in the early 1980s, studying the disease was not enough. Researchers focused their attention on the immunological system in the body to see how the virus was affecting people. From that research, they were able to develop treatments that eased the worst AIDS symptoms. Thanks to their hard work, an AIDS patient today can enjoy a longer and richer life.

Today, the NIH has 27 institutes and centers that study all areas of medical science. Researchers and doctors from all over the world work with the NIH. Since 1977, the agency has held what they call Consensus Development Conferences. Scientists from around the globe gather to discuss their work at these meetings. They may talk about a new disease, a new cure, a new medication, or a new method of performing an operation. They discuss their research and try to come to a group agreement. If, for example, several of the scientists and doctors at the conference have found that a certain medication is working well in treating a disease, they may all agree that it will become the medical standard. If Dr. Kinyoun were alive today, he would most likely be astounded at the worldwide collaborative effort that grew from the small beginnings of his one-room Hygienic Laboratory.

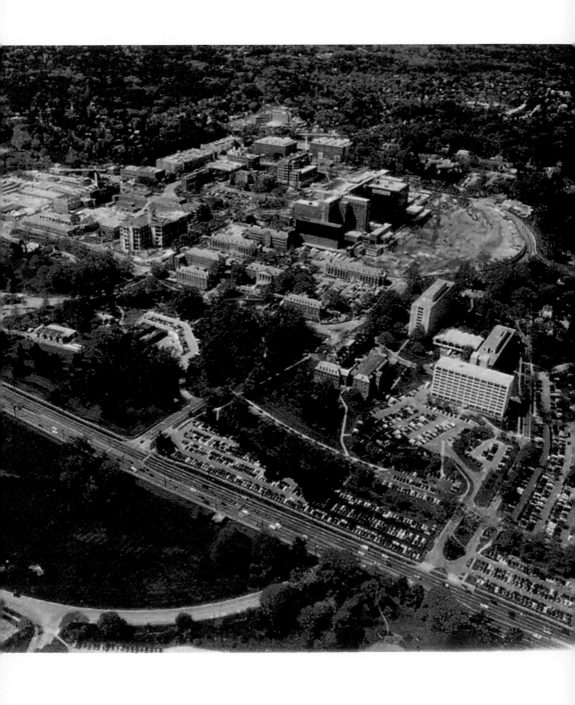

CHAPTER **3**

The NIH Today

TODAY, THE NIH is one of the most important research centers in the world. Part of the U.S. Department of Health and Human Services, it is the leading medical research center in the United States. The NIH main headquarters is in Bethesda, Maryland, just a few miles from the capital of Washington D.C. The NIH campus includes 75 buildings on 300 acres (121 hectares) of land. Research conducted on the campus is called **intramural** research. Several NIH off-campus facilities and field stations are also considered part of the intramural research programs. About 10 percent of the NIH budget goes toward intramural research. The remainder is designated for **extramural** research programs, with grants going to projects around the world. Both intramural and extramural research programs focus on the same goal: to help prevent, detect, diagnose, and treat diseases and disabilities.

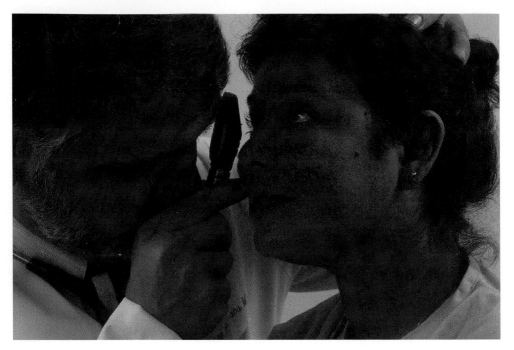

The mission of scientists at the National Eye Institute, one of the many institutes that make up the NIH, is to conduct research that will protect and prolong the vision of the American people.

The Institutes

Twenty-two institutes and several centers and offices make up most of the NIH. Each of these organizations receives money from the government to study a different area of science and medicine. Combined, the institutes, centers, and offices conduct research on thousands of projects in their labs and provide millions of dollars to universities, medical schools, hospitals, and research institutions to pursue their own research.

The National Eye Institute, for example, studies any illness that can affect a person's vision. Scientists conduct research on cataracts, glaucoma, and other eye-related problems and diseases. The National Eye Institute has helped develop such advances as medical lasers to treat eye diseases and correct vision. Researchers have also developed safe and effective drugs to treat a variety of eye ailments.

The National Institute on Aging studies how the body changes as it grows older. Scientists there look at diseases that may affect people at different stages of life, when they turn 50, 60, or 70 years old. In addition, researchers study ways to help people stay healthy as they grow older. Scientists at the National Institute on Aging are working toward finding new treatments for conditions that generally affect the elderly, such as Alzheimer's disease, arthritis, and osteoporosis. Their goal is to help everyone enjoy a longer, healthier life.

The National Institute on Alcohol Abuse and Alcoholism is another example of the many institutes that make up the NIH. Here, scientists conduct and support both medical and behavioral research on the causes of alcoholism. They look at the effects of alcohol on the body and study the damage it can do to fetuses during pregnancy. Researchers seek ways to prevent and treat alcoholism and conduct studies to figure out which groups of people are more likely to have problems with alcohol. This institute also works to spread the word to the public about the dangers of abusing alcohol.

In some cases, more than one institute will study the same disease. For example, Alzheimer's disease, which usually affects older people, attacks the brain and has a great effect on memory, thinking, and behavior. Because the disease is related to aging, mental health, and the brain, it is studied by the National Institute on Aging, the National Institute on Mental Health, and the National Institute for Neurological Diseases and Stroke.

Other Facilities

The NIH includes several facilities that support the research efforts of the institutes. Among them are the Center for Information Technology, the National Library of Medicine, and the DeWitt Stetten, Jr. Museum of Medical Research. The Center for Information Technology not only provides the computers and networks needed for conducting research, but also identifies new computer technologies that can be applied to medical research. The National Library of Medicine, which is the largest medical library in

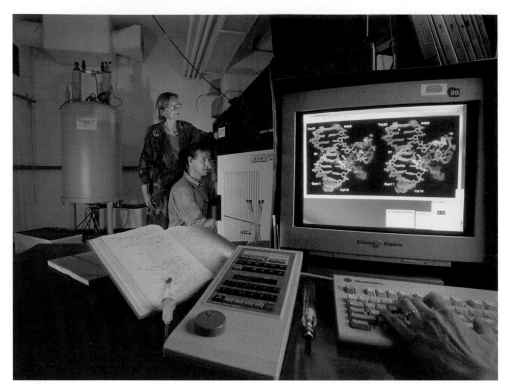

Scientists examine molecules using a high-powered scanner and computers. The Center for Information Technology helps identify computer-related technologies that can aid scientists in medical research.

the world, has helped develop a medical library network with 4,000 hospitals and other facilities. The library also offers an extensive Internet site to provide scientists, health care workers, and the public with medical information. The Stetten Museum was established in 1987 as part of the NIH's centennial observance. The staff there collects medical research instruments and prepares exhibits to explain how medical research is conducted.

One of the most important buildings on the campus is the Warren Grant Magnuson Clinical Center, a combined research hospital and laboratory. Unlike most hospitals, this center does not treat patients who come in with illnesses. Instead, the hospital is devoted to conducting clinical research. The patients in this hospital are there to be part of research studies or experiments. The Clinical Center's goal is to use laboratory discoveries to create effective treatments. A brand new facility, the Mark O. Hatfield Clinical Research

Center, is scheduled for completion in 2003. It will provide more space for conducting NIH clinical trials.

NIH Grants

The NIH has a budget of more than $20 billion to support its medical research, both on the NIH campus and in other facilities around the world. Extramural researchers apply for grants to pay for their medical research. But not every medical research scientist who wants a grant gets one. Scientists, doctors, and researchers send in applications to the NIH main offices asking for funding for their work. Each application explains what will be studied and why the research is important. Some researchers seek a cure for a disease currently affecting many people. Other scientists looking for funding hope to find ways to prevent future illnesses. Still others want to learn more about how the human body works. From rare diseases to the common cold, research grant requests cover all kinds of diseases and health conditions.

The NIH reviews as many as 38,500 applications for research grants every year. Choosing which medical research projects to investigate is not an easy decision. No single project, research laboratory, disease, or doctor has priority over others. Although some new diseases appear that need immediate attention, diseases that have been around for some time still need study to find treatments.

For each field of research, the NIH puts together a group of top scientists to help decide which projects should receive grants. These scientists try to select the research projects that will contribute the most to fighting disease and providing new information about health. A project such as studying human genes, for example, does not help in preventing one disease, but it may help doctors get a better idea of how the human body works. This knowledge might then lead to prevention of many diseases. Sometimes a project may sound rather odd, such

NIH scientist Christian Anfinsen accepted the Nobel Prize for chemistry in 1972. In all, 97 scientists associated with the NIH have won the Nobel award.

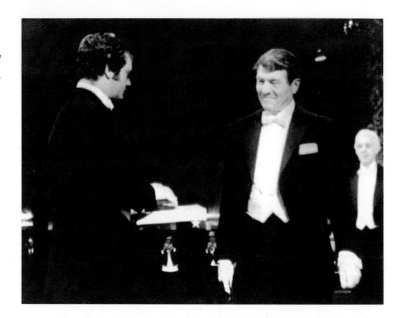

as studying a type of plant or the cells of a certain animal. If you know, however, that the drug penicillin, which treats infections, was created from mold or that the vaccine that cured smallpox came from cowpox, anything is possible when it comes to medical science. Therefore, if the scientists or researchers who want a grant have shown that there is good reason to believe that they may make progress in fighting a disease, even if it sounds unbelievable, they may receive a grant.

The NIH's intramural scientists, as well as those who have received grants, have made many exciting discoveries and have also worked diligently day by day toward better means to diagnose, prevent, and treat diseases. Over the years, 97 of these scientists have won the Nobel Prize, the greatest honor awarded for science. Five of these Nobel Prizes have been won by NIH scientists who work in intramural laboratories.

Spreading the Word

Years of scientific research have provided the NIH with a great deal of knowledge. As part of its mission, the NIH

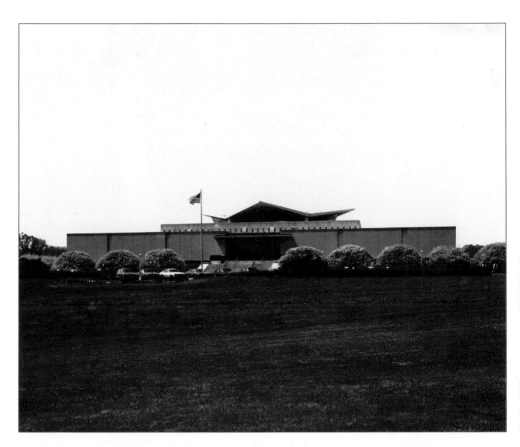

works to communicate information about their successes, and even their failures, so that the medical world and the public will have the latest information about the prevention and treatment of diseases.

To help spread the word, the NIH has created a comprehensive Internet site that has the latest information and statistics about thousands of diseases. The site contains links to each institute, where information on their research and clinical trials is available. Details on nearly 10,000 medications can be found through a link to the National Library of Medicine. The site also provides a look at the organization of the NIH and states the key goals of each institute as well as the goals of the organization as a whole.

The National Library of Medicine on the NIH campus is the world's largest medical library.

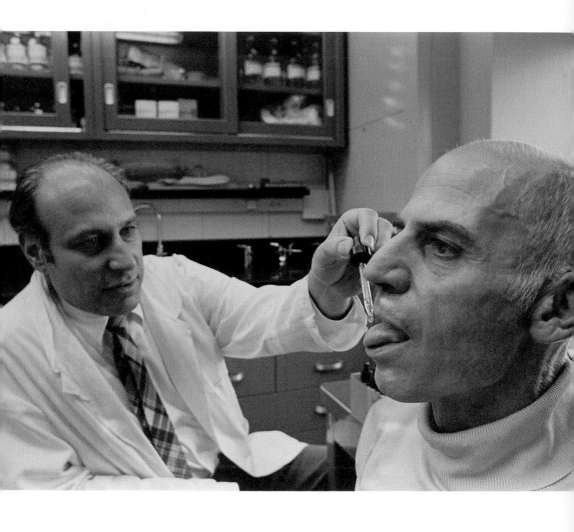

CHAPTER 4

Clinical Trials

THE NIH SUPPORTS thousands of research projects every year. New discoveries about how the body works, new ways to detect disease early, information about the effectiveness of new treatments, and new ways to prevent diseases are the results of the many hours scientists spend working in their laboratories. Because all the work is being done to help people stay healthy, the final—and one of the most important—steps in the NIH research process is the clinical trial, which tests medicines and treatments on people.

Protocol and Criteria

There are many rules to make sure that no one who participates in a clinical trial is in danger. The rules used during a clinical trial are called a protocol. The protocol describes the type of tests and medications that will be included, how long the clinical trials will take, and which people can be included in these studies. Clinical trials have guidelines for who will be allowed to take part. If you apply for a clinical trial, for example, researchers will carefully study your medical history. The scientists and doctors will look at which illnesses you have had and which medications you have taken. Clinical trials do not include only people with illnesses. People who are healthy also take part, allowing the scientists and doctors to compare the results between healthy and sick people.

If you are allowed to be part of a clinical trial, the reasons that allow you to be included are called inclusion criteria. For example, if the trial needs someone who has no allergies and you have no allergies, then the fact that you don't have allergies is a reason you would be included in the trial. The reasons that keep you from being allowed to participate are called exclusion criteria. For example, if someone were allergic to the medication that is going to be used in the study, then that allergy to the medication would keep that person out of the clinical trial.

Informed Consent

Before a clinical trial begins, the NIH must have what is called informed consent from every person who will be involved. Informed consent means that someone has learned all the facts about the clinical trial before deciding whether or not to participate. These facts include why the research is being done and what the researchers want to accomplish. Researchers should also explain exactly which medicines participants will take during the trial or what types of treatment will be given. Participants should know, too, what benefits to expect from the trial and that they have the right to leave the trial at any time. Participants need to understand that the medicines or treatments they receive may or may not help them. The goal of a clinical trial is not to help an individual, but to gather information that will help the larger population.

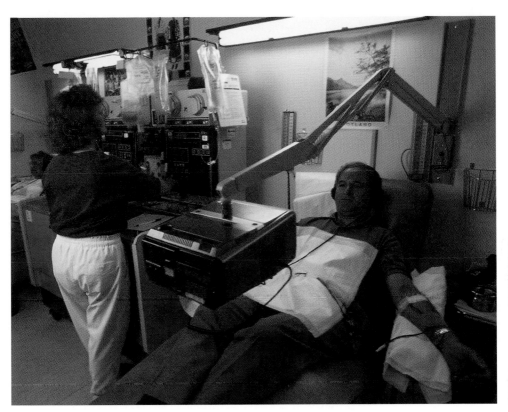

While part of the study, each person is monitored by the research staff. It is important to make sure someone does not become ill from the trial. Committees of doctors also get together to make sure that the rights of all people involved are protected. These committees watch over the clinical trial to make sure that each participant knows exactly what is being done and why.

A man donates blood platelets at the NIH's Warren Grant Magnuson Clinical Center. The platelets may be used in clinical studies involving blood transfusions.

Phases

Like most scientific experiments, a clinical trial has several parts. The different parts of a clinical trial are called phases. In the first phase, the new medication is given to a small group, usually fewer than ten people. Researchers use this phase to make sure the medication will not harm people, and they look for side effects.

Then the researchers move to phase two in which they

give the medication to a slightly larger group, usually about 100 people. Researchers use this trial to determine dosages, deciding whether it is best to give people more, less, or the same amount of the medication that they gave to the group in phase one. They study whether the medication is working to cure the illness or condition, and they continue to watch for side effects. They also compare whether the medicine is helping to cure the condition or illness in a way that is better than other types of treatments.

Phase three of the study is testing the medicine on a large number of people, sometimes as many as several thousand. By this time, the researchers are confident that the medicine is safe, but they continue to look for additional side effects and how the medication is working to treat the illness.

Finally, in phase four, the drug is approved to sell in pharmacies. Doctors can now **prescribe** it, and it is considered to be "on the market," or available to whomever needs it. The researchers then look to see what the effects of the medicine are over a long period of time for the people who were in the clinical trials. It is possible that after the drug is available to the larger population, other side effect may emerge that were not found during the clinical trials.

Control Groups

Some people who take part in the phases of a clinical study are not given a new medication at all. For an experiment to be successful, scientists need to compare what they are testing against current medications. For example, people usually take aspirin to get rid of headaches. Let's suppose that you, as a scientist, have just created a medicine that you think will work better than aspirin. But the only way to be sure it will work better is to compare the two. Therefore, if you were allowed to do a clinical trial, you would give your new medication to one group of people and aspirin to another group. The people taking aspirin would be called a control group, because they are taking the usual

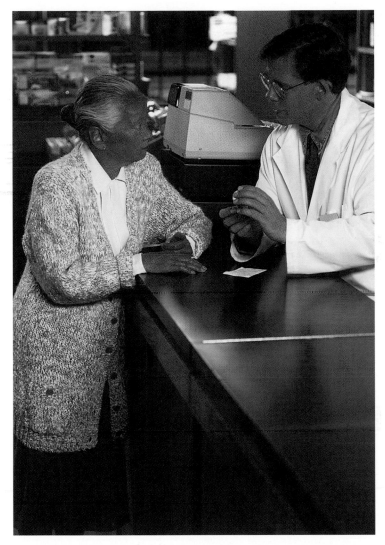

During phase four of a clinical trial, a new medicine is available for doctors to prescribe. Pharmacists help make sure patients know the correct dosage to take.

cure or treatment for a headache. You would then watch the two groups to see if your medicine got rid of the headache faster than the aspirin and if it had any side effects.

In clinical trials, people are divided into two groups. One takes the new medicine or treatment and the other, the control group, takes the usual medicine or treatment. In some cases, a control group is given no real medicine at all. They receive what is called a placebo, a pill or liquid that does nothing. With this approach, researchers can see if a

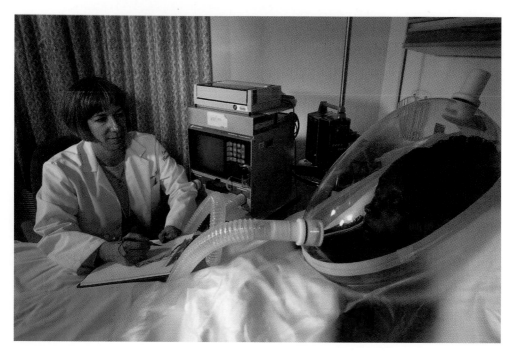

A researcher conducting a study on kidney metabolism observes a woman using a breath analyzer. Researchers make sure clinical trial participants receive good care throughout a study.

medication will help or if no medication is necessary at all. Sometimes a completely different type of treatment, such as exercise or a better diet, is found to be more helpful than a new medication.

Participants usually take part in blind or masked studies in which they do not know whether they are taking a new medication, an existing treatment, or even a placebo. Some studies are even double-blind or double-masked experiments. In these studies, neither the participants nor the researchers know which people are receiving the test treatment and which are getting standard treatment or a placebo. Both types of studies are meant to discourage participants' and researchers' expectations from influencing the outcome.

Benefits and Risks

The NIH has conducted thousands of clinical trials. The hospital facilities at the NIH are designed to inform people about clinical trials and to conduct the research. People taking part in these studies are often those you will find in this hospital, along with the doctors, scientists, and research assistants.

For the people who take part in clinical trails, some will be the first to benefit from new medications or receive expert treatment before the general public, usually without spending a lot on medical bills. They will be cared for by top medical experts. But some participants will not benefit at all, other than being paid to be part of the experiment. Others will experience side effects or bad reactions to the medication, possibly without any positive effect on their overall condition. But the benefits usually far outweigh the risks when you consider the broad application of clinical trial outcomes. NIH scientists and doctors gain valuable information about medications that may eventually treat thousands of people effectively.

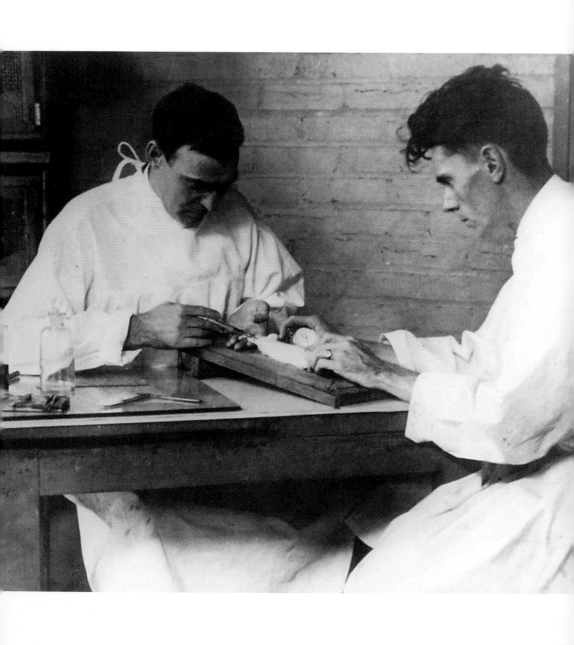

CHAPTER **5**

Scientific Breakthroughs

FOR MORE THAN 100 years, government scientists have been working to find treatments for diseases, to learn about the human body, and to apply their knowledge to better the health of Americans and people everywhere. Through experiments in laboratories and clinical trials, the NIH has played an important role in many important scientific **breakthroughs** and discoveries.

Early Discoveries

Back in 1902, for example, a team of researchers set out to investigate a disease called Rocky Mountain Spotted Fever. The disease, which was also known as black measles, was killing people and there was no cure. Headaches, a rash, mental confusion, and a high fever occurred in people who had the illness. In 1906 scientists discovered that the disease was caused by the bite of a tiny bug called a tick. In 1921, researchers opened a laboratory in Montana to help study and fight this disease. They were able to develop a vaccine to keep people from dying from the disease. Today, Rocky Mountain Spotted Fever still exists, but it can be easily treated with medications.

Another breakthrough was in the battle against pellagra, a disease that causes a skin rash and mouth sores, and once often resulted in death. In the early 1900s, pellagra was widespread across the southern United States, mainly affecting the poor. The Public Health Service sent Dr. Joseph Goldberger, one of their leading doctors, to the southern states to investigate the terrible illness.

Goldberger discovered that pellagra was caused not by a germ, as people thought, but by the corn-based diet of many poor Southerners that lacked **nutrients.** This idea was not readily accepted by the general population. So Goldberger set out to prove his case through a study of eleven prisoners in Mississippi. Some prisoners ate a balanced diet of fresh meat, vegetables, and milk. Others ate a corn-based diet. Sure enough, in a few months, the prisoners eating the corn-based diet showed symptoms of pellagra, while the other prisoners remained healthy.

Still not convinced, many Southerners continued their regular eating habits, and pellagra continued to ravage the South, killing 10,000 people in 1921 alone. It wasn't until an infestation of boll weevils killed most of the cotton crop that Southerners were forced to diversify their crops and grow more vegetables. The change in crops also changed the Southern diet, and cases of pellagra dropped. Later researchers discovered that pellagra resulted from a deficiency of vitamin B. Goldberger's work was a major step in showing how important the research of the Public Health Service was not only for contagious diseases but for nutritional and **chronic** diseases as well.

Recent Discoveries

NIH researchers have made many other important scientific discoveries that affect all of us. In recent years,

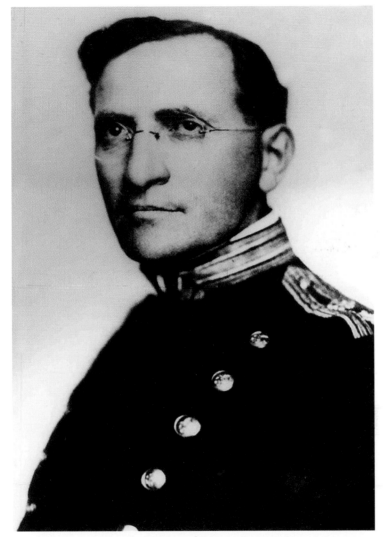

Dr. Joseph Goldberger investigated the causes of pellagra, an often fatal disease that was widespread across the southern United States in the early 1900s.

scientists have created detailed maps of the human brain that show how it develops. From this work, researchers have discovered, for example, that people best learn new languages before the age of 12, when growth in the region of the brain that controls language begins to slow down. In other studies, scientists proved that not getting enough sleep can be harmful not only to the mind but also to the body, making it easier to develop some serious health conditions such as diabetes and high blood pressure. Researchers also

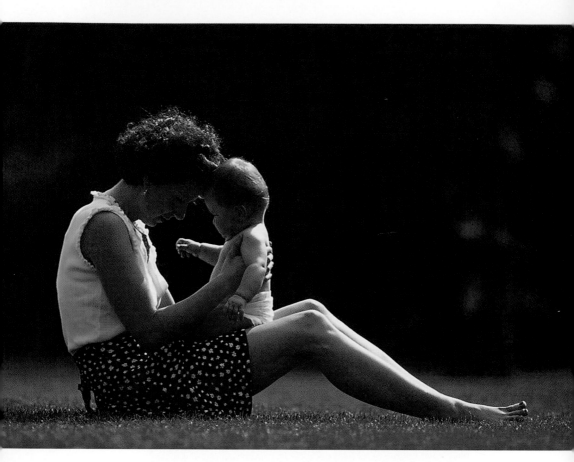

Passed from parents to children, genes not only determine how people look but also the illnesses they might get. Scientists at the NIH hope that their work on gene research will lead to breakthroughs in treatments for inherited diseases.

discovered the role of high **cholesterol** in heart disease and how it is possible for many people to control the level of cholesterol in the body through diet and exercise.

One of the most important current research programs at the NIH is the Human Genome Project. Genes determine all the different traits and characteristics of each person. For example, genes will determine if someone is going to be tall or short, have brown eyes or blue eyes, have straight hair or wavy hair, or be shy or outgoing. Genes can also pass illnesses, or the possibility of getting an illness, from one generation to the next. For example, if your mother had gum disease, you might have the same gene in you that could cause problems with your gums. Knowing this in advance, you could see the dentist more often, floss frequently, and take other precautions so that you won't inherit the same gum disease.

Understanding human genes is like having an instruction manual for people that also tells what makes them different from each other. The research at the NIH and around the world has already led to a new understanding of genes and how they affect our health. It shows us which diseases and illnesses are passed on from parents to their children. Scientists believe that there are as many as 4,000 different diseases that children can inherit from their parents. Knowledge of these specific genes is the first step in finding ways to cure inherited diseases.

These breakthroughs are only a few of the many examples of important research work done by the NIH. Scientists have little time to focus on all that they have accomplished, however. They must continue to explore new diseases and work toward gaining new knowledge about treatments for existing diseases.

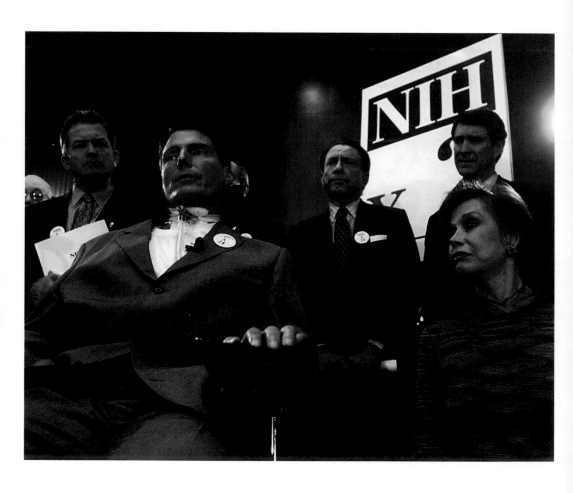

CHAPTER

6

The NIH in the New Century

IN MAY 2001, NIH Acting Director Dr. Ruth Kirschstein appeared before House and Senate subcommittees to present the NIH budget request for 2002. She acknowledged the support of the president, Congress, and the American people in providing additional funding. " . . . Progress in the medical sciences is advancing at a speed we only dreamed of a few years ago," she said. "This is a time of extraordinary opportunity." And indeed, the beginning of the 21st century has brought seemingly limitless potential in advancing scientific knowledge and applying that knowledge to the prevention, treatment, and cure of diseases and health problems.

Present Dangers

Doctors and scientists will need to address new health threats while continuing to battle existing diseases. One of the biggest medical

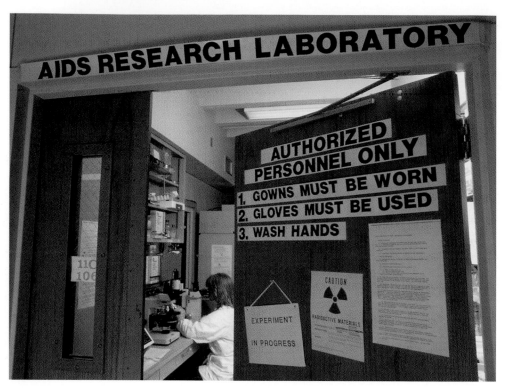

This AIDS research laboratory is part of the National Institute of Allergy and Infectious Diseases.

concerns today and for the future is HIV and AIDS, which continue to spread without a known cure. The Office of AIDS Research is dedicated to researching this deadly disease, which attacks the body's immune system.

Congress has funded the Office of AIDS Research, authorizing its scientists to organize all AIDS research efforts throughout the United States. This research includes seeking out a vaccine against AIDS, as well as a cure. It also includes studying both people who have been infected with AIDS and those who are at risk of being infected. The NIH supports 100 locations throughout the country that conduct clinical trials on new drugs. It also supports research programs to create a vaccine to protect the immune system against infection. The fight against AIDS, a disease that has already killed millions of people, is one of the toughest battles for the NIH.

Bioterrorism is a real threat to the United States and

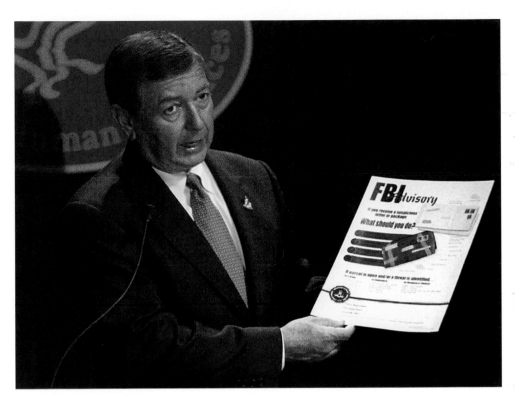

another major concern of the NIH in the new century. Bioterrorism means spreading chemicals or disease-causing microorganisms with the intent of harming or killing people. In the fall of 2001, shortly after terrorists attacked the World Trade Center in New York and the Pentagon in Washington, D.C., the United States was faced with bioterrorism for the first time. Government officials and the news media received envelopes in the mail containing anthrax, which are dangerous bacteria. Anthrax, which can be deadly if inhaled, had not appeared in the United States for many years.

Attorney General John Ashcroft discusses an FBI advisory about the deadly bacteria anthrax in October 2001. The diseases that could result from bioterrorism will be a major focus of the NIH in the coming years.

The Federal Bureau of Investigation (FBI) followed the trail of the anthrax-filled letters. Investigators worked to put together evidence in hopes of finding out who was behind this terrorist act that killed several people and made others ill. The NIH teamed with several other federal health organizations, such as the Center for Disease Control and

Prevention, to provide treatment advice and to answer the millions of questions from people around the country who called to learn more about symptoms of anthrax.

But scientists were not fully prepared for the anthrax attacks. Although they had been familiar with anthrax for more than 80 years, they were not very familiar with the military type of inhalation anthrax that was spreading through the mail. NIH scientists had to work quickly to learn all they could about this type of anthrax and the medications needed for effective treatment of those who had contracted the disease. The spread of anthrax through the mail also caused NIH doctors and scientists to start preparing in case smallpox and other illnesses that have not been seen in many years also return through bioterrorism. Doctors must be able to test people for these diseases and have the drugs on hand to stop an epidemic.

Another very different manner of spreading disease will also be of major importance in the coming years. Because diseases can be passed down from parent to child, a great deal of attention will continue to be given to the Human Genome Project and its eventual effect on all areas of medicine. Larger teams of scientists, including specialists in chemistry, biology, mathematics, computer science, and statistics are now joining the research scientists to study genes more closely. Doctors and scientists are hoping that the Human Genome Project will become a guidebook for the human body in the 21st century and will have long-term effects on medicine and healthcare. Knowing which genes can carry which illnesses will make it easier for scientists and doctors to fight diseases.

Technology and Communication

New medical technology will also continue to be very important to the work of the NIH. Many new computer programs are helping doctors and scientists record and analyze the data from their experiments and studies.

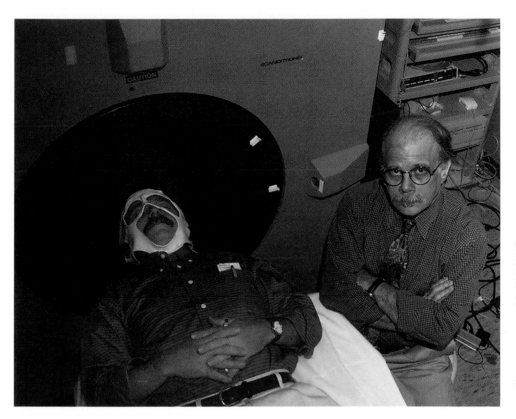

Advances in medical technology are also making it easier to diagnose illnesses. For example, advances in a technology called body imaging allow doctors to see a picture of how the body is functioning. And researchers are working hard to improve body imaging techniques even more.

The need for clear and accurate information about medicine and health grows every day, and the NIH is dedicated to providing this information to medical workers and the public. The NIH and the many NIH institutes are constantly adding to their web pages so that individuals can look up illnesses and learn about the latest medical research.

New technologies in body imaging will aid in the research of NIH scientists. Here, a researcher is using positron emission tomography scanning (PET scan) to study changes in the body during sleep.

The Future

A hundred years ago, scientists could not have imagined the leaps and bounds that medical science took in the 20th century—from a vaccine against polio to a survey of

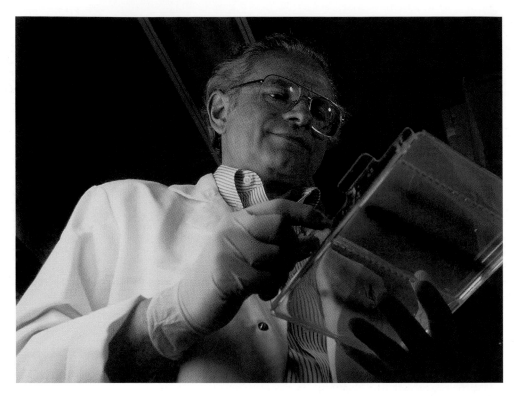

An NIH researcher works on a type of DNA map. The mapping of the human genome, one of the most important projects at the NIH, could be the key to treating and preventing many diseases.

the human genome. Today, NIH researchers look to the future optimistically in search of new breakthroughs and discoveries.

Experts see the mapping of genes as the key to solving many medical mysteries in the 21st century. Scientists are working to compare human genes to those of other organisms, such as mice, fruit flies, and monkeys. These comparisons will help them identify which genes cause human diseases. Researchers are also looking at what they call modifier genes, or those human genes that influence how a disease-causing gene works. Pinpointing these modifier genes will tell scientists, for example, why there are differences from person to person in the way a disease progresses. With these approaches, researchers hope to identify genes involved in causing cancer, heart disease, diabetes, Alzheimer's, and many other diseases and then find effective treatments and cures.

NIH scientists hope that their current research will lead to other breakthroughs. A focus on global health, for example, could lead to new vaccines that would eliminate such epidemics as tuberculosis and malaria. Advances in neuroscience research may help patients with brain injuries or spinal cord injuries recover fully. Researchers may find new ways to stop a body from rejecting transplanted organs. Doctors may be able to screen fetuses in the womb for genetic disorders and then correct the problem before a baby is even born. Scientists may even find ways to grow new tissue from a patient's own cells. A newly grown artery, for example, could be used during heart surgery. Researchers also hope that helping parents educate children about staying healthy will prevent the onset of diseases as they grow into adults.

The role of the NIH and other government agencies has expanded far beyond what the Founding Fathers could have imagined when they established the Constitution in 1787 to, in part, promote the general welfare of the people. Armed with increased government funding, new technologies, dedicated scientists, and the ability to communicate its findings, the NIH is equipped to carry out this mission in the new century.

NIH Institutes, Centers, and Offices

National Cancer Institute

National Eye Institute

National Heart, Lung, and Blood Institute

National Human Genome Research Institute

National Institute on Aging

National Institute on Alcoholism and Alcohol Abuse

National Institute of Allergy and Infectious Diseases

National Institute of Arthritis and Musculoskeletal and Skin Diseases

National Institute of Biomedical Imaging and Bioengineering

National Institute of Child Health and Human Development

National Institute on Deafness and other Communication Disorders

National Institute of Dental and Craniofacial Research

National Institute of Diabetes and Digestive and Kidney Diseases

National Institute on Drug Abuse

National Institute of Environmental Health Sciences

National Institutes of General Medical Sciences

National Institute of Mental Health

National Institute of Neurological Disorders and Stroke

National Institute of Nursing Research

National Library of Medicine

Center for Information Technology

Center for Scientific Review

John E. Fogarty International Center

National Center for Complementary and Alternative Medicine

National Center for Minority Health and Health Disparities

National Center for Research Resources

Warren Grant Magnuson Clinical Center

Office of AIDS Research

Office of Behavioral and Social Sciences Research

Office of Dietary Supplements

Office of Rare Diseases

Office of Research on Women's Health

Glossary

Bacteria—The smallest of microscopic organisms; bacteria are single-celled organisms.

Breakthrough—A sudden advancement in knowledge or a technique.

Cell—The smallest part of an animal or plant.

Cholesterol—A type of fat made by the body that can clog arteries in the heart and lead to heart disease.

Chronic—Always present or reoccurring.

Clinical research—To take a discovery made in a laboratory and apply it to practical use by testing on animals and humans.

Contagious—Able to catch from someone else; contagious diseases can pass from person to person very quickly.

Extramural—To function outside an organization; the NIH gives grants to extramural researchers who work in their own hospitals or laboratories.

Genome—The entire genetic material of an organism.

Hygiene—To establish and maintain good health.

Infectious—Capable of causing infection.

Inflation—A general increase in prices.

Intramural—To function inside an organization; intramural scientists work directly for the NIH in its laboratories.

Microscopic organism—A living being that can be seen only through a microscope.

Molecule—The smallest part of a substance that contains all the chemical properties of that substance.

Nutrient—Something that is needed to stay healthy; vitamins and minerals are examples of nutrients that people need.

Prescribe—To order the use of a medication or other remedy.

Sequence—A set of elements arranged in a certain order.

Side effects—Effects caused by a medication other than treating the illness for which you are taking the medicine. For example, if a medicine to make your sore throat go away also makes you sleepy, then being sleepy would be the side effect.

Vaccine—A medication that prevents a person or animal from catching a disease.

Virus—A tiny microorganism that reproduces and grows inside living cells and that causes diseases.

Further Reading

Altman, Linda Jacobs. *Plague and Pestilence: A History of Infectious Diseases.* Issues in Focus. Springfield, N.J.: Enslow, 1998.

Anderson, Laurie Halse. *Fever 1793.* New York: Simon & Schuster Books for Young Readers, 2000.

Aronson, Virginia. *The Influenza Pandemic of 1918.* Great Disasters and Their Reforms. Philadelphia: Chelsea House Publishing, 2000.

Bottone Jr., Frank G. *The Science of Life: Projects and Principles for Beginning Biologists.* Chicago: Chicago Review Press, 2001.

Dennis, Carina, and Richard Gallagher. *The Human Genome.* New York: Palgrave, 2001.

DeSalle, Rob, Ed. *Epidemic! The World of Infectious Disease.* New York: The New Press, 1999.

Hyde, Margaret O., and John F. Setaro. *Medicine's Brave New World: Bioengineering and the New Genetics.* Brookfield, Conn.: Twenty-First Century Books, 2001.

McPherson, Stephanie Sammartino. *Jonas Salk: Conquering Polio.* Minneapolis: Lerner, 2002.

Storad, Conrad J. *Inside AIDS: HIV Attacks the Immune System.* Minneapolis: Lerner, 1998.

Websites

The official Website of the National Institutes of Health: *[http://www.nih.gov]*

The Website of the Dewitt Stetten, Jr. Museum of Medical Research: *[http://www.nih.gov/od/museum]*

Index

ABOUT THE AUTHOR: Rich Mintzer is the author of 26 nonfiction books, including several for children and teens. He has also written articles for national magazines and material for high school students for the Power To Learn website. He has been a professional writer for nearly 20 years and enjoys writing on many different subjects. Rich currently lives in New York City with his wife and two children.

SENIOR CONSULTING EDITOR: Arthur M. Schlesinger, jr. is the leading American historian of our time. He won the Pulitzer Prize for his book *The Age of Jackson* (1945) and again for *A Thousand Days* (1965). This chronicle of the Kennedy Administration also won a National Book Award. Professor Schlesinger is the Albert Schweitzer Professor of the Humanities at the City University of New York and has been involved in several other Chelsea House projects, including the REVOLUTIONARY WAR LEADERS and COLONIAL LEADERS series.

Picture Credits